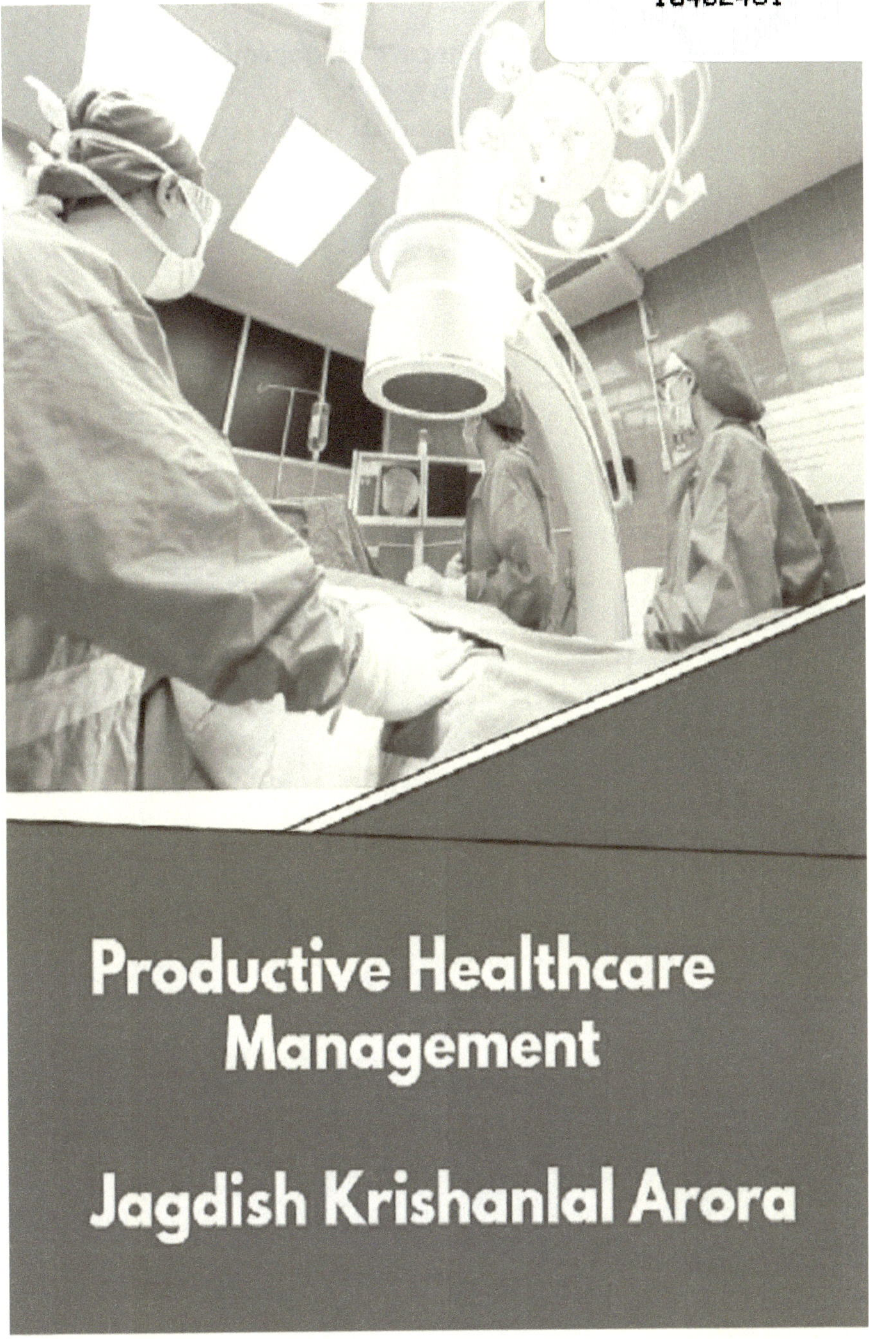

Productive Healthcare Management

Jagdish Krishanlal Arora

Productive Healthcare Management
By
Jagdish Krishanlal Arora

While every precaution has been taken in the preparation of this book, the publisher assumes no responsibility for errors or omissions, or for damages resulting from the use of the information contained herein.

PRODUCTIVE HEALTHCARE MANAGEMENT

First edition. February 2, 2024.

Copyright © 2024 Jagdish Krishanlal Arora.

Written by Jagdish Krishanlal Arora.

Table of Contents

Title Page

Copyright Page

Chapter 1: Introduction

Chapter 2: Collaborative decision making through shared governance

Chapter 3: Administrative ethics

Chapter 4: Conceptual frameworks: Ethical constructs of ethics, moral or legal standards

Chapter 5: Medical disclosure and secrecy

Chapter 6: Treatment costs

Chapter 7: Marketing and business plan processes for DNP – Doctor of nursing practice

Chapter 8: Understanding financial challenges

Chapter 9: Medication error reporting and disclosure

Chapter 10: Ethical, moral and legal dilemmas in treatment

Chapter 11: Recruitment and training of healthcare professionals

Chapter 12: Insurance and claims

Chapter 13: Diagnostic testing

Chapter 14: Child development observation and parental care

Notes

Sign up for Jagdish Krishanlal Arora's Mailing List

Further Reading: How to Lose Weight Quickly

Also By Jagdish Krishanlal Arora

Chapter 1: Introduction

THE PROPER STUDY OF healthcare systems is necessary to improve the quality of healthcare. The authors try to combine the knowledge from study of healthcare improvement measures with existing literature. Existing improvement measures for a few foundations are studied by using existing systems for meeting the initial requirements and integrating them with future requirements with the help of literature to find appropriate solutions.

The major challenges identified in improving healthcare are in asking people to believe in the issues that is relevant to them, convincing them with a right solution to that problem or issues, using that solution, collection data and monitoring the solution, projection, identity, categorize the solution, staff engagement, leadership roles and risks of implementation and results.

The author identifies a range of tactics that may be used to respond to these challenges. The healthcare solutions face many challenges and proper study of these problems and their solutions are needed to address them. With increasing focus on safety of patients measures to improve healthcare show improper results due to the difficulties to implement the solutions. The large number of healthcare programs work to improve quality of health with no obvious results. Main challenges faced by healthcare systems.

1. Convincing people there is a problem and finding the

right solution.

2. Collecting proper data.

3. Analyzing the data with past and present events.

4. Projections with likely improvements that can be

achieved.

5. Convincing the healthcare employees to implement the solutions from the perspective of the patients as well as for the betterment of the organization is hard and difficult considering the Suo motto nature of the programs.

Healthcare employees are always skeptical about the solutions and it is the same with the patients due to unintended consequences if things go wrong. Having more and more focus on automation and getting things done with the help of machines healthcare has a long way to go where both the healthcare employees and the targeted beneficiaries to get proper care and treatments and make them at ease. This also requires a cost and the benefits are immense in the long term.

Chapter 2: Collaborative decision making through shared governance

COLLABORATIVE DECISION making is a necessary requirement and an operational system which helps to make important decisions between the management and the staff. In Medicare, nursing provides the necessary base and infrastructure to organize the delivery of care and through shared governance nursing integrates the practices and core values for achieving quality care. Shared governance practices have improved the working environment and satisfaction of employees and provides better governance and employee retention.

Shared governance framework

Shared governance is reliable and has lived up to its expectations and potential and provided the much-needed returns for good governance. The model of shared governance is a form of a political system in an institution and balances power between the different constituents and gives the platform required to build a consensus. Although, conflicts are common in labor management, these can be better managed through shared governance, which provides the necessary space to negotiate and bargain for the proper function of the institution and provide the necessary services, especially in health care where co-operation is very important in-patient care and wellbeing, and any conflict arising may affect the treatment of patients. In healthcare and Medicare there are three parties involved the management, the nursing staff and patients and all the factors must be considered while delegating responsibilities and duties or sharing them so patient care is not affected by conflicts of interest.

Implementation through participation using shared governance

Shared Governance system developed by nurses who worked at a facility created a system focusing on accountability and unified decision making. They create a model of care taking, making the nurses accountable and allowing other staff members to attend meetings and promote timings and setting agendas. The agendas involved multitasking and maintaining discipline in the system and could be used in the entire organization to maintain excellent care. The model is a success and increases staff engagement and can increase participation to 60-70 percent from 30-35 percent before implementation of the system and gives encouraging results. There are clear goals set for the shared governance system which could measure the progress and eventually achieve implementation and fosters competition for giving quality services.

The four elements in shared governance hold the nurses accountable, focusing on the task at hand, implementing them and having an open communication within the system. There is a focus on patient satisfaction and building a leadership team to boost patient care and offer training for nurses. Success in using shared governance is to increase the safety of patients, educate the staff and increase employee awareness and growth in our organization.

Conclusion

Healthcare professionals are positioning themselves in the market to strategically remain at the top and need shared governance to remain ahead of competition and provide better healthcare services than others in the market. Shared governance models include Herzberg (1966) and McGregor (1960) who favored employees as an organization's important asset and encouraged organizations to invest in employee growth and motivation. Deming (1986) introduced the new concepts of quality management and suggested that work environment should be modified to improve quality, empower workers to produce more and focused on leadership and team building. Gardner & Cummings (1994) and Thrasher et al. (1992) said forms of shared governance was formed in alliance with an organization's quality management decisions. The various types of shared governance are decided to be decided by committees at different organizational levels, dividing decision making, authority and participations between different people within the organization depending upon their level of importance within the organization. (Bereuter, 1993).

Governance through self-managed teams

An alternative to a shared governance system is governance through self-managed teams. They are very much like self-governance but have the additional benefit of having leadership to manage and supervise decisions. Leadership roles are important and responsibilities in a self-managed team have additional responsibilities and this is different from traditional teams, which are based on hierarchy. Self-management means long term goals and development as well as personal development of the team members. In traditional teams the roles of the members are vested in one individual, but in self-managed teams, each member can contribute significantly by providing support and coaching to the other members in the team, through counseling, advice or contributing to the work involved directly.

In traditional teams' instructions are given from top to bottom and the top management acts only for giving orders or minimum directions and the results may be positive or negative depending on the capabilities of the down staff who carry out the instructions. There are several benefits of self-management as it involves well-defined tasks and instructions. In a traditional team, it is left to the discretion of the employee to provide the results or fail, resulting in delegating the responsibilities to other alternative employees/employers.

Self-management results in moral support where the employees are trusted to do the job without any outside interference. (Richard Y. Chang & Mark J. Curtin, 1999). In self-management the individuals have the chance to prove their capabilities which is not possible in the traditional system.

In a traditional system the tasks are delegated based on employees post and not on the capability of the person to carry out the job. Instructions are monitored in traditional management for completion and in self-management the purpose is only to see the task completed and handed over to full satisfaction. (Cloyd Hyten, 1997). There are substantial savings involved with self-management as it reduces employees and additional requirements of supervision and employees with lower qualification who carry out the tasks can prove their working skills. Team members are given a chance to improve their working styles and practices in line with the requirements. This gives better productivity and the turnaround time is faster. Work gets done quickly due to saving in time in passing out the instructions from one employee to another. The team has a common goal, and this results in roughly 25 % more productive than traditional teams and they do not have to wait for instructions from higher ups. This helps improve customer services and sales of the organizations due to lower complaints as instructions from higher ups is not needed to act on urgent matters.

All members of a self-managed team share equal responsibilities for completion of the project resulting in lesser blame shifting on other team members for inefficient work done. This reduces stress and disputes between the team members.

There are also problems associated with self-management, which include no proper culture and individuals working on their own may go astray and other members may not get to know about ongoing projects unless they are actively involved in the day-to-day functions. Individuals may complete the tasks without informing the other members if they are absent and this may result in duplication. The possibility of duplication of work may not arise in traditional management. For those members need to be aware of other team members work in a self-managed system. Therefore, in self-managed teams proper planning is required and team members need to coordinate with each other and maintain proper communication. There should be trust between different team members and one individual cannot supersede the other individual in the team in a zeal to complete the work on his own without help from other team members. (Cloyd Hyten, 1997). For the self-managed teams to work better would require proper coordination as well as a friendly interaction between different team members resulting in optimum performance. In self-management the leaders should be changed from time to time as keeping one person as a leader would hinder improvement and leave the organization solely in the hands of one single individual. Over a period, the individual may feel his place secure and will result in a drop in operational management and no new ideas will come up for the benefit of the organization and the system. Leaders also tend to become arrogant and slow listeners if not replaced with time.

Chapter 3: Administrative ethics

ETHICS IS VERY IMPORTANT in life and is applicable to all activities that we do. Being ethical improves reputation and work life, installs a sense of self-esteem, respect, rules and regulations and building trust and to be ethical is to be trustful and reliable. Ethics plays an important role in defining services offered by Healthcare Systems. If the services offered are honest, in line with the disease and actual cost of treatment is given then the Healthcare System is believed to be Ethical in fulfilling its responsibilities to society. Ethics, also known as moral philosophy, addresses questions about morality and what is good, evil, right or wrong, justice and crime. The ethical values help us to judge right or wrong under the circumstances and the corrective action that need to be taken.

All organizations involved must declare that the treatments carried out by them are honest and justified in protecting the health of the patient and necessary for his survival or wellbeing and be affordable. Ethics is very important in life and is applicable to all activities that we do. Being ethical also improves our reputation and work life, and installs a sense of self-esteem, respect, rules and regulations and makes us trustful and reliable. International council of Nurses has released a guide "ICN Code of Ethics for Nurses" for action based on the social needs and values. Administrative ethics is concerned with influencing the behavior and ethics of their members, behavior of members in the organization, and with each other and overseeing if the rules and regulations to be followed by the members as well as the organization.

The work of administrative ethics also includes following the guidelines laid down by the government, obeying the laws of the land with respect to the organization and dealing of its members and organization with the community and government. This means that the implementation of decisions by the providers should consider the values and ethical behavior of its members in line with existing laws as well as rules of the organization should be followed especially in the care of patients to be a successful provider.

The National Center for Ethics in Health Care's was founded in 1971, headquartered in Washington, DC administers various fields which include medicine, nursing, philosophy, law, policymaking, education, theology, social work, and health care administration.

The activities and initiatives of the organization include support for clinical ethics, organizational ethics, and research ethics and VHA's National Ethics Committee provides analysis and guidance on controversial ethics issues affecting patients, providers, health care managers, and health policymakers.

To deal with ethical issues an organization must be comprehensive, establish clear standards, roles, competencies, methods, and performance metrics for its members and the patients. It should have a multi-level, multi facet program supported by a national policy, sophisticated training programs, validated evaluation tools and a robust communications network.

The leaders of the organization should be accountable through specific targets in their performance plans and requires continuous monitoring and quality improvements. It should also provide the much-needed assistance to patients, families, and staff and deal with any eventually that might have occurred. The organization must provide patient rights and provider rights, have commitment to quality and standards and have a moral duty towards those being served in line with laws and regulations.

The HIPAA Privacy Rule provides federal protections for personal health information held by covered entities and gives patients' rights to the information and the

privacy rule is balanced so that it permits the disclosure of personal health information needed for patient care and other important purposes.

The security rule specifies a series of administrative, physical, and technical safeguards for covered entities to use to assure the confidentiality, integrity, and availability of electronic protected health information.

We all believe that our medical and health information is private and should be protected. The privacy rule is a federal law which gives rights over our health information and sets rules and limits on who can look at and receive your health information and it applies to all forms of individuals' protected health information in the electronic, written and oral form.

The security rule protects the health information in electronic form, and it requires entities covered by HIPAA to ensure that electronic protected health information is safe and secure.

The entities covered include all health plans, insurance companies and government programs that pay for health care, health care clearing houses and entities that process nonstandard health information they receive from another entity and health care providers that conduct certain business electronically including doctors, clinics, hospitals, psychologists, chiropractors, nursing homes, pharmacies, and dentists.

To maintain the patient's confidence, the physician should not disclose the medical information revealed by a patient or discovered by a physician during the treatment as required by the AMA's code of medical ethics.

The physician has an ethical and moral duty to ensure patient confidentiality if the patient has passed on full information about his illness and related factors. Since the disclosures enable the physician to diagnose the illness and offer proper treatment, full confidentiality is necessary to protect the information which is sensitive and may affect the patient's image and wellbeing in society.

This information should not be passed on without the patient's consent unless required to disclose the information by law. There are some exceptions to the rule in case of self-injuries and in case where a physical harm is done to others etc.

The managers and healthcare professionals must behave in an ethical way and use the information in a diligent way. This is especially true in case of celebrities and high-profile people and politicians for example in the case of Michael Jackson who was had a history of medical problems and diagnosed with a rare disease at the time of death. Since the information about his condition was of a very sensitive nature, information about his medical condition was to be protected at all costs.

In that case the HIPAA rules could not be considered restriction of information to his family or friends and the rules permit doctors or other health care practitioners to share information that case is directly relevant to the involvement of a spouse, family members, friends, or other people identified by a patient.

Therefore, if the patient has the capacity to make health care decisions, the doctor can discuss this information with the family or others present if the patient agrees or when given the opportunity and do not object to the disclosure.

The doctor may in this case share this information with family members or friends when, in exercising professional judgment, the doctor determines that doing so would be in the best interest of the patient. This is proved by the fact that the nursing profession is always in an ethical dilemma to maintain privacy and to justify them. There are several ethical decisions to be made as to the disclosure of information and the implications and legal consequences. This involves moral values as well as responsibility towards the organization and the profession which needs to be justified in decision making. For the managers and physicians these issues involve social responsibility, ethical values and duties.

For an organization the protection of information is very important as being a provider and the success of the organizations and systems in which they work, but in ethical terms the recipients of services should get appropriate privacy and protection.

Michael Jackson's November 15, 1996 marriage to Debbie Rowe, a former nurse, age 37, took place at a hotel suite in Sydney, Australia. She knew Jackson for 15 years before they were married and was apparently six months pregnant at the time of their marriage and had to sign a confidentiality agreement stating that she couldn't speak to the press or anyone in the public about "Michael, the children or our lives together."

In protection of private information physicians and healthcare professionals need to consider ethical and social responsibilities and not all providers are influenced by such

ideals and it is rare that providers, managers and physicians take these into consideration while deciding on the health needs of the patients.

The decisions of protection of private information are closely interrelated because, health care professionals are responsible to themselves, the boards in case of an organization, patients to whom they provide service and a moral obligation to society in which they live. In case of a misfire or failure to do so may result in legal implication and litigation.

The personal physician of Michael Jackson had to stand trial for involuntary manslaughter after hearing testimony that he administered a lethal dose of a powerful anesthetic and other sedatives then left the pop star alone and the ruling in the case against Houston cardiologist

Dr. Conrad Murray came after a six-day preliminary hearing before Superior Court Judge Michael Pastor.

Prosecutors concluded their case with testimony from two doctors who said Murray acted outside the standards of medical care.

THESE FACTORS ARE PARTIALLY controlled by being accountable; limits imposed by the organization rules but, the result of such regulations lies solely with the providers and the ethics of the organization as well as the healthcare professional.

However, it is to be seen that if the regulations are indeed effective to ensure that the best interests of the public, organization, professionals and shareholders is taken care of in protecting privacy. In other words, the healthcare professional has a duty towards the organization, the patient, third party payers, government, shareholders, and community and to himself for all aspects of his decision and administrative ethics.

Ethical conflicts related to privacy and disclosure of information may be created with the agency or within an organization or due to outside factors. The conflicts can be addressed through proper understanding of the conflict and the factors that caused the conflict to take place.

The solutions to resolve the conflict are done by finding the nature of the conflict, clarifying wherever necessary, proposing verification, using alternative methods and taking preventive and corrective measures to end the conflict and action.

Chapter 4: Conceptual frameworks: Ethical constructs of ethics, moral or legal standards

DUE TO ADVANCES IN medical technology, political and social changes result in moral dilemmas for both patients and physicians. This in turn creates conflicts for nurses. (Martin Benjamin, 2010 p. 1). We are very fortunate to have a variety of ethical theories which provide support for making ethically correct decisions and solving difficult issues.

Ethical theories take the support of ethical principles which help to decide what is right or wrong, when trying to reach the best decision. When one understands each individual theory, and its strengths and weaknesses, decisions can be taken when trying to achieve an ethically correct answer to a dilemma. Developing a balanced approach to ethics with an emphasis on the positive benefits of ethics and development of a good character is good, and there are positive advantages of being ethical and negative results of being unethical.

The primary purpose of ethics is to take the right decisions and is the medium for the development of a person's character to use the knowledge to benefit him and others.

The National Center for Ethics in Health Care was founded in 1971, Washington DC and administers various fields including medicine, nursing, philosophy, law, policymaking, education, theology, social work, and health care administration. The activities and initiatives of the organization include support for clinical ethics, organizational ethics, and research ethics and VHA's National Ethics Committee provides analysis and guidance on controversial ethics issues affecting patients, providers, health care managers, and health policy makers.

Constructs of ethics

Ulrich et al. (2010) studied the nature of ethical issues faced by nurses and it was seen that more than 60% of nurses said that the patient's right to autonomy, and consent was the cause of frequent problems faced by them.

The other issues were decision making, advanced care planning, confidentiality and end-of-life decision (Ulrich et al., 2007. It was found that ethical issues, actions and regrets of nurses resulted in pain and suffering, delinquency in patient autonomy and difficulty in decision making. To solve these problems the nurses communicated and spoke up by advocating and collaborating (Pavlish et al., 2011).

CONSTRUCTS OF MORAL standards

To deal with ethical issues an organization must be comprehensive, and establish clear standards, roles, competencies, methods, and performance metrics for its members and the patients. Everyone in the organization should be accountable through performance plans and require continuous monitoring and quality improvements, providing the much-needed assistance to patients, families, and staff and deal with any eventually that might have occurred.

The organization must provide patient rights, have committed to quality and have a moral duty towards those being served in line with laws and regulations.

Many companies have an ethical policy and employees need to be trained to follow the policy defined by the organization. The government must bring in regulations to make it compulsory for Healthcare Systems to have an ethical policy as is there in the case of many public listed companies who have their own ethical policies for their employees.

CONSTRUCTS OF LEGAL standards and high cost of treatments

The most common issues affecting health care and the patients are the high costs of health care and the payers like third party insurance companies are more than less willing to take on the burden of various procedures and in some cases legal issues. There is a scarcity of resource allocation decisions both by managers and physicians, and with limited financial, technical and knowledge resources, equitable and appropriate distribution has become necessary.

This is where administrative ethics come into play as it provides the moral decision-making tools that individuals, organizations and communities need to determine and justify the norms and structure the terms under which scarce resource allocation decisions are required to be made to balance costs.

The cost of healthcare equipment is high for the sole reason that the equipment's are costly. The prices are at a premium for the sole reason that the equipment's are being used to treat patients who are willing to pay whatever charges the hospitals demand for their treatments.

Margins and profits are high in purchasing or selling of healthcare equipment's. This needs to be balanced. Lowering cost of purchase of equipment will result in lower cost of treatments of patients.

The cost of training and education is also high as Universities and Schools of medicine procure instruments and equipment's are high costs leading to increase in the cost of education. Therefore, only a limited number if schools of medicine have necessary infrastructure for medical students.

Having actual treatment equipment's for schools of medicine is not necessary and some schools of medicine also offer treatments in addition to teaching to make it practical for students to learn while they are studying in the college. This balances the cost of equipment and can also offer cheaper treatments for those in need.

Ethical, moral or legal dilemma encountered in the workplace Healthcare professionals may in the name of technical expertise impose their professional values on others without justification (Martin Benjamin, 2010 p. 12) Most of the time therapists face ethical and moral dilemmas while treating patients and must ponder on the legal and ethical values before treatment.

Not all patients are financially stable and most borrow from relatives and friends to cover the cost of treatments because they are very high. Had the treatments been affordable, there would be less financial hardship for the patient and encourage him to go for treatment.

Many patients prefer to suffer agony and pain as the treatment specified is not correct and is only done to prolong the illness as a recurring income for the Healthcare provider.

Many healthcare providers give delayed treatment and make patients sit in hospitals waiting for the expert doctors to arrive and diagnose before treating them.

While the patients wait for the availability of the doctors, they are put under the supervision of nurses or local staff and the treatments do not start but the billing by the hospital continues for the stay without attendance by a doctor who is most of the time busy with other patients.

Even after a doctor arrives, he seldom comes occasionally to go away quickly to treat another set of patients in another hospital. Because of the limitations of the hospital to employ a full time doctor whose cost is too high to bear, the hospitals often rely on part time visits by other specialists who are often over occupied with work and have more than enough to handle.

ETHICAL POLICY

Money cannot be the sole purpose of treating patients as while the patients are in hospital they are in acute need of proper treatments and that is why they are in hospitals. It is agreed that specialists are limited but hospitals can always keep a full-time local doctor to take care of patients until the specialist arrives. The cost can be recovered by offering good services and patients often come back or recommend to others if they get good services.

It is good to specify to the patients the treatments available and recommend to them an honest cure. Many a times patients go away to other hospitals if they find the hospitals do not have the necessary support of doctors or specialists or the necessary equipment's for treatment.

This is because other hospitals with full time doctors and proper equipment convince the patients that their services are superior than those offered by hospitals with poor infrastructure and lack of hospitals.

With increasing cost of specialists and normal doctors now even big hospitals are unable to afford them full time and only keep nurses for full time services. Lower cost hospitals keep only staff and no doctors and no nurses to manage costs. Nobody can be blamed, and it is only circumstances that affect such situations.

The priority of hospitals should be to lower costs and when it lowers its cost of operation, the cost for treatments will automatically go down. Making money is a priority for doctors, specialists and hospitals but it should be reasonable and affordable for the patients.

If you have too many patients you cannot handle, offer the excess to other doctors and specialists. It is not humanly possible to attend all patients only by one specialist or doctor or one hospital. If we have many patients, we need more hospitals to foster competition and this helps in improving services and lowering costs of treatments.

In one case the hospital had a very big building housed with doctors round the clock. It offered the best of the facilities and running costs were also high, but it used ordinary iron pieces fitted for treating knee problems of patients. The patient never came to know that he was implanted with low quality iron fittings in his knee until the iron started to corrode, and it appeared as brown patches in his legs.

This hospital spent most of the money in paying for staff, nurses, doctors who were paid a commission for referring patients and to specialists who carried out the treatments. The patients were happy while in hospitals only to know the consequences later when it was too late.

Also, the hospital was owned by an owner of a big company who hardly had time to attend to seeing what his hospital was doing and how it was running as it was only a charitable hospital dedicated to the memory of his mother. It was more for publicity rather than treatment still the cost charged to the patients was abnormally high which only the rich or the affluent ones could afford. People went to the hospital as a matter of prestige rather than treatment to say that they received treatment in a hospital whose owner was part of a large enterprise.

For small treatments the hospital was good like any other local hospital but still cost was high even for ordinary ailments. For larger operations the hospital used substandard parts and spend most of the money in services of doctors and infrastructure costs.

While the hospital looked good from outside attracting patients its operation efficiency was hidden by its huge building and staff and services. The hospital did not focus on providing quality treatment but provided only a big infrastructure to make it look impressive.

If we recall, army people are treated on stretchers, in the jungles and in times of war people are treated on roads and on the wayside by only nurses with no doctors or specialists and still survive grave wounds.

They don't get big hospitals and beds and ICU units but still many survive and recover. Big buildings are necessary, but the focus should also be on quality treatments.

Chapter 5: Medical disclosure and secrecy

MANY HOSPITALS HAVE secrecy, means that neither can the treatment be specified neither the cause of illness and other such things. This is because patients and their relatives do not have medical knowledge and it would be too vague for them to understand medical terminology and diagnosis of illness.

The hospital has no declared guidelines for either informing the patients or their relatives about the illness, treatment required or the treatment costs and the duration of the treatments. This secrecy is different from that which is transferred to public domain to newspapers and other such agencies and is related to the actual treatment and its costs.

IF NOT TALKED ABOUT the illness, the patient does not know what his illness is and why is he being treated at the hospital and why is he being operated upon. If not possible to inform the patient it should be informed to the relatives taking care of him. Treating a patient without knowledge of illness either to him or his relatives may be a ground for an offence or a legal action.

Some hospitals take an undertaking before start of a treatment that the patient is aware of his illness and has agreed to the treatment being carried out fully with his knowledge and in case, he is incapable to understand the persons accompanying him for treatment are taken into confidence before the start of a treatment.

If not part of the Ethical policy this needs to be part of the guidelines on how a hospital or a doctor treats a patient to cover his costs of operation or to cover both his costs as well as provide treatment. Sometimes patients are kept indefinitely just for sake of earning money or to cover costs of operating the hospitals. This needs to be investigated in more detail.

But most lower hospitals explain everything to the patients or their relatives but since they have no facilities recommend them to higher hospitals. The patients or their relatives going along with them for treatment sometimes accept those suggestions offered by the lower hospital and go to the fully equipped hospitals having the necessary facilities for treatment. But the premium hospitals hide the illness details and often give a muddy or a vague picture of the treatment required. The patient has no choice once admitted to either carry out the treatment or pay for the brief stay of diagnosis.

Chapter 6: Treatment costs

TREATMENT COSTS ARE generally not affordable for everyone except the premium class and even for some of them it is heavy. They even generally prefer visits by home doctors as it is cheaper to them. But the premium or high value paying customers are only 1-5 % of the total patients depending from hospital to hospital.

But if patients could be diagnosed for an illness at home by sending doctors or specialists at reasonable costs to the home of the affected patient it would lower costs and make more beds available for treatment to other needy persons.

While premium patients get diagnosed at home by either personal doctor visits by specialists the poorer patients get no such facilities.

The home visit facilities should also be provided to poorer patients as it would save them costs and it is seen that most poor patients are lured into being admitted without having the necessary financial support.

The patient should only be admitted in hospitals if treatment was affordable to him and the diagnosis would be honest as the healthcare system would-be aware the patient can cross check with other providers if the diagnosis given was correct or not. In case home based service is not possible healthcare institutions must try to lower their cost of operations.

Many healthcare institutions do not want to lower costs as due to this they see a surge in the amounts of patients coming to them when their costs become cheaper than others.

A higher costs limits people to come to a hospital and all these aspects must be investigated to find the best option to lower costs as well as avoid sudden surge in patients rushing for treatment. A home-based option may help to avoid overcrowding at hospitals.

Home based services to lower the cost of healthcare

It is desirable to lower the costs of healthcare, we should now start providing home-based services which would be easier to handle and maintain. If the hospital has lack of staff this can be made as a separate unit which operates independently of the regular services in the hospitals.

Very few people operate in these areas and those are not yet approved fully. But with so much strain on existing hospitals and no beds availability and lack of

specialists, staff and doctors and nurses a home base solution would be an ideal option.

Industry has already started making equipment's which are compact and can diagnose many illnesses with home-based equipment's. This initiative for home-based services will also foster invention in making equipment's which are smaller in size and can treat patients at home avoiding, if possible, the necessity of an operation or help to diagnose a disease in the early stages.

Hospital based services face many challenges which include lack of parking facilities. Priority for parking is for hospital employees, the doctors, nurses, ambulances and outside specialists leaving little or no space for vehicles of patients or relatives even after having big hospital space.

Patients have only beds and there is not sitting areas for relatives as most spaces are occupied by doctor rooms, nurses and so no and no toilet areas are there for visitors either. All these hurdles can be overcome by providing home based services especially for illness which are too small to be treated in hospitals. More the 80 % of the illnesses are not critical and therefore require no hospitalization. But sometimes we find in such minor cases patients are in hospital but patients with critical illness get left out as the hospitals have no beds available.

Often hospitals advise patients to get admitted for normal cases due to which beds can unnecessarily occupied and when an emergency case comes up there is no space for those cases.

The hospitals need to keep a percentage of the beds reserved for such cases and need to shift patients or discharge patients early who are either sitting in bed or can recover at home instead of occupying precious pace required by critical patients who need urgent hospital care.

Chapter 7: Marketing and business plan processes for DNP – Doctor of nursing practice

SWOT ANALYSIS - STRENGTH, Opportunities, Weakness and Threat

Using SWOT analysis, the DNP can find the advantages, by providing innovative solutions and saving in costs. This can be done by looking for new opportunities, improving profits through innovations, and identifying threats from existing competitors in the market who provide superior services.

The weaknesses include the absence of a proper marketing plan, ageing equipment and facilities, and poor service quality. The DNP should be properly trained in care, and focuses their attention on bedside nurses, with the ability to provide moral support, to take care of the diverse

needs of the population by providing a supportive work environment (Murphy, Stepileno and Carlson, 2015).

This can be done by acquiring knowledge and skills to create a practical environment, to develop a cordial patient nurse relationship and care. This training should also be provided by the healthcare institutions to the healthcare professionals from time to time.

This creates a better health care system to provide patients, with human caring values and life purposes, as opposed to only the economics of treatment for purely monetary benefit.

By collaborating with other nurses and using them as partners to deliver change, and provide the necessary professional support, to improve the system is also necessary. DNP specialists generally do not have direct patient care responsibilities and practice at the system or organization level but are sometimes called to give solutions on solving health care issues as and when they arise.

Through the proper use of collaboration facilitates, there is a transformation from research into practice, which can drive positive change and enhance educational opportunities and improve healthcare facilities.

The different knowledge and skills that the DNP has provided an opportunity to collaborate to conduct research and improve practice environments (Edwardson, 2010).

Chapter 8: Understanding financial challenges

HEALTH CARE PROFESSIONALS face financial challenges to ensure that their billing and coding departments bill and code properly for receiving payment from various healthcare payers. DNP must ensure the use of proper billing and coding specialists, mostly outsourced and certified and the DNP needs to understand the financial impact the system act accordingly (Dreher & Glasgow, 2016).

The Leadership provided by DNP depends on developing a cordial relationship with fellow nurses and shape policies in the best interests of patients at the micro level.

The DNP should be capable of providing proper analysis of health policies with patients, other fellow nurses, and healthcare professionals taking into consideration the interests of these stakeholders in the middle level or mesosystem.

The strategy includes considering the local, state and federal and corporate and international issues of health policy at the macro level system, since these factors influence the policy makers, and are utilized in research to shape health care policy initiatives at the local, state, federal and committee levels. The education programs for nurse's face difficulty to prepare enough nurses to fulfill the vision to provide a better US healthcare system, and to ensure that a enough highly trained nurses are available to work, practice and research,

The best practices include using professional collaborations and use of the domestic and international service work and working with the to change the system as per required and bring about the desired improvements in the system.

Implementation is important to bring about the desired change in the DNP program through various research polices at the organization level (Anderson, 2014).

Chapter 9: Medication error reporting and disclosure

MEDICATION ERROR, TREATMENTS and corrective measures

Human errors do occur, and identification of errors is very important. These medical errors can occur with nurses as well as physicians and registered nurses should be familiar with the occurrence of medication error and their disclosure and identification.

An error requires clarification after it has been detected and it requires corrective steps to be taken and to ensure patient safety. Most errors occur due to improper communication or to carry out treatments in a hurry.

Some errors occur as the instructions given are inadequate to the lower staff often due to busy schedule or a rush of customers or unqualified supporting staff. The

decisions made in such a situation have moral and personal implications. (Arndt, 1994)

Scenarios

Most of the errors which occur are related to prescribing a drug to a patient and it is not intentional but could have adverse effects on the health of the person. If the error has been detected corrective action needs to be taken to prevent further damage.

But it is very difficult to disclose the error as it may have lots of legal and other implications and disturb the patient who may take it otherwise. Ethically, it is the right thing to do, but if the patient does not agree with the explanation provided, he may take legal action.

However, if the nurse or the physician can explain the health concerns, and how the harmful effects can be minimized, in a proper way, and why they occurred, it may provide a solution. Giving an apology is the best thing to do and possibly avoid its recurrence in the future. (Cohen, 2006).

Normally, patients will be satisfied with an apology and you can explain to try and rectify the error, rather than the patients finding it out later. The best remedy is how you handle the situation, by reporting the error and taking corrective action, as soon as it is discovered rather than waiting for an explanation.

In practice. Nurses are responsible for reporting all errors, irrespective of the consequences involved. Errors can be reduced by devoting enough time to each patient, as errors occur mostly due to insufficient time, and many

patients were treated simultaneously, resulting in a mix up in medication in different patients with the differentiation diagnosis. Lack of time also causes errors in giving the wrong medicines, to the wrong patients as there is a hurry to attend them mostly in emergencies.

Errors may also occur in both oral as well as written prescriptions. Written prescriptions should have details of the person's name on them. Oral instructions for patients should be avoided as far as possible, as this may be the most likely causes of errors.

When prescriptions are given without a name on the prescription paper, it may lead to medication error. (Cronenwett, Bootman et. Al., 2007). Other types of medication errors also include giving too much dose of a medicine or prescribing the wrong medicine for an ailment which does not exist.

Painkillers are the most common medicines give for many kinds of reliefs and taking too much of them causes harm to the important body organs. Some medication errors occur due to a high dose and in severe cases, too low, a dose may also lead to serious implications and the disease aggravation.

The side effects of the drug also need to be considered and the resistance of the patient to the drugs prescribed and history and lifestyles of the patient also need to be investigated. The patient may need to be informed about the side effects of the drug, so he is aware of them. (Davis, 1981)

Conclusion

It is very important, how the medication error is handled, and disclosure is the right thing and to ensure proper rectification and apply the necessary measures at the right time.

Many physicians say they are open to any errors that may have occurred, but the reality is they do not disclose them and often cover them up or try different ways to hide them before they get known to the patients.

Chapter 10: Ethical. moral and legal dilemmas in treatment

PRACTICAL EXAMPLE OF an ethical, moral and legal situation and its analysis

Take an example of a female patient who was on alcohol for some years and a mother of two children and wanted treatment to solve her drinking problem. She had stopped drinking for a few months but received news that her company was on verge of closing and may file for bankruptcy.

The patient had started drinking again and appeared for the therapy session drunk and had even abused her children due to the pressure. As the therapist was in two minds whether to treat her or report her for abuse.

In the first instance, it appeared that the patient should be treated and if she responds positively, then as a therapist, he should ignore the legal implications and other factors. In this case the ethical conflicts occurred due to outside factors.

Analysis of the moral, ethical and legal implications utilized in the specific situation

In the above case of the female patient on alcohol, the conflicts were to be addressed through proper understanding of the conflict and the factors that caused the conflict to take place. The solutions to resolve the conflict was done by finding the nature of the conflict, clarifying wherever necessary, proposing verification, using alternative methods and taking preventive and corrective measures to end the conflict and action in this case being alcoholic.

Ethical dilemma involved

It required giving into a client's request as the patient who would otherwise quit therapy and it would not solve the problem. The second issue was that it would make the client depend on you or if termination of the therapy was the most suitable option to take.

Moral dilemma involved

It showed a desire for the negative feelings towards a client due to the situation and feeling upset over it. This also showed that the client's moral values were different from my own and the client's character was something which was disliked and resembled those people whom we would like to avoid in life.

There is also a question of autonomy and respect of personal information which the client has shared, and they

have the right to live their lives provided it does not harm others, particularly in the case of counseling by mental health experts making the treatment viable and client safe from external and legal implications.

Legal dilemma

Here such factors come into play, which include our emotions and vulnerabilities, and therefore influence our decision-making process on how to deal with patients in such situations. It is not always possible to help each client, but the goal is that if the patient is treated properly, he may not cause harm to his children or abuse them.

Sympathy

We should also be courageous and kind towards our patients making them feel welcome and complete the

treatment in hope for a better and healthy life both physically and mentally.

Results of diagnosis

Moral implication

Such cases mostly take place in mental health problems where most patients need to get over their bad habits and need the help of mental health therapists where secrecy is of most importance.

Ethical implication

In such cases we need to be sympathetic to the patient, so treatment of the patient is of utmost importance in such cases. The Charter in Medical Professionalism states that professionalism demand placing the interest of patients above those of the physician and setting and maintaining standards of competence and provide expert advice to society on the matters of health (Albert R. Jonsen, Mark Siegler, 2015 p. 14).

Legal implication.

If secrecy is broken treatment of the patient is not possible and legal remedies would only aggravate the problem. Legal implications would only be an alternative if the patient did not respond to treatment or was unwelcoming to treating himself which was not a factor in this case.

Leadership style: Identified as a barrier or facilitation in the dilemma

Leadership Style as a Barrier in the Dilemma

Not taking the problem of the patient seriously would only aggravate the problem and act as a barrier and considering the legal implications would only make matters worse and would be a hindrance to treatment as the patient may have been subject to accusations of abuse and alcoholism.

Leadership Style as a Facilitation in the Dilemma

Facilitation the treatment if available and providing the necessary moral support would enable the patient to overcome his bad habits and improve his quality of life. The patient will also take the treatment steps to improve his quality of life and avoid further abuse of his children in the future.

Conclusion

The patient was genuine in his case to solve the problem and had himself approached the therapist to get himself treated and if such treatment is available the best course would be to continue treatment of the patient till the problem is resolved to the satisfaction of all concerned. The best solution in this case would be to treat the patient and help him and the society in general.

Chapter 11: Recruitment and training of healthcare professionals

THIS STUDY IS FOCUSED on the evaluation of key considerations of individuals joining the healthcare profession and their selection which include doctors, nurses and other staff. It focuses on the experiences and challenges faced by these new professionals, prior to their registration and considers the importance of the social aspect of the healthcare profession and focus on training and acquiring the necessary skills.

It also considers the problems faced in maintaining the individual identity, in a professional context at the commencement stage of professional life.

Aims and objectives

Individual experience at a certain level in such professions is highly affected by organizational culture, employment opportunities, regional and demographic dynamics, and the relative importance of the field in society. The aim of this discussion is to provide a crucial insight into the effective and practical implications of the research, and to evaluate the effects of changes experienced, during a transition from academic to professional life in healthcare.

However, it is observed from the description of the aims and objectives that the study has been structured loosely, in relation to the context of the research (Holloway & Galvin, 2017).

The research titles also suggest a wider framework that includes additional considerations like professional progression, industry and economics, and a wide variety of other dynamics, not only on the experience of the individuals on a personal level. The paper focusses its attention on key issues relating to the considerations being evaluated and discussed.

Methodology of the Study

The study uses Interpretative-Phenomenological-Analysis (IPA) as a primary methodological basis. This method is based on the presumption that there is a correlation between the actual experience and individual perception and emotional responses. The study uses a qualitative basis for the research and interviews.

The sample size taken for the purposes of the study consists of eight students with only one male participant from a batch of graduates and was conducted through telephonic interviews using a tailored form of the original IPA approach. The time span was twelve-month period and the methodology emphasized on the input from professionals who had knowledge and experience with the subject matter (Naylor, Ferris, & Burton, 2015).

The study employed one key qualitative technique for obtaining data. The IPA may be used for identification of key theme on certain levels, that have been experienced by several individuals, but due to the lack of structured approach and guidance it has been causing problems on the application level (J, J, E, & C., 2011).

One of the key pre-requisites is the level of skill and competence of the person, conducting such interview, along with the awareness that researcher's personal dispositions. These factors have been accounted for, from the IPA technique of the previous applications, and the quality of outcomes largely depends on the attention and quality of feedback from participants.

The interviews largely took place over phones and may put the quality of inputs and feedbacks from participants into the question, as the circumstances of those individuals at the time of phone call are largely unknown and not accounted for (F, et al., 2014).

The sample selection method does not use any statistical approach, and no estimations have been used as to the sample size, and its relation to population size.

Furthermore, it has been observed that the sample must be representative of the overall population, using IPA. Consultations with professionals and practitioners with previous experience relating to the use of technique, and subject matter, adds to the credibility of the study.

Findings in the context of relevant literature

Findings suggest that the transitional period of academic life to professional one has significant impact for individuals in healthcare profession, and due to existing and emerging situations, it is characterized by challenges and opportunities.

The study reflects the importance of academic institutions to prepare students for these challenges, as the current system has not been accounting for the same. The study also concludes that experience-based learning along with theoretical support plays a crucial. It also emphasizes on the importance of a supportive environment, for freshly employed individuals and has been found to have a positive correlation with transition process effectiveness.

An effective transition process allows fresh graduates to align themselves with the profession's needs and the environment in a better way, than if the same transition was to be ineffective. Finally, this paper emphasizes on the need for further work on cultural aspects and its implications.

Additionally, a study of the same variables in different professional settings may also be helpful in providing useful insight into more facts relating to the subject matter (Naylor, Ferris, & Burton, 2015).

Summary

The aim of the study can be structured and tested. The aims and objectives have been loosely structured and research titles suggest a wider framework It has been successfully able to focus its attention on key issues and employs one key qualitative technique for obtaining data (IPA).

It assesses key pre-requisites for the application of the method being employed and sample selection method and statistical approach are used. The study has successfully integrated the results of key findings and conclusion and recommendations are satisfactorily being drawn in connection with the requirements.

It may be observed from the structure of these conclusions, that there is a strong coherence in a continued pattern, and the study has successfully integrated the results of key findings by addressing each aim defined for the purpose. (Elo, et al., 2014).

However, the study has not been able to incorporate the cultural and other major environmental aspects that fall under the scope of the study and have been discussed in the methodology. Thus, it may be argued that the conclusion and recommendations are satisfactorily being drawn in connection with the requirements and context of the study with few exceptions.

Selection and Recruitment process for healthcare professionals. It is seen healthcare professionals are hired indiscriminately without proper recruitments and procedures followed and there is hardly any recruitment

checks involved and considering it as a profession of trust people are often hired as a matter of trust rather than on experience and actual requirement.

Those who work on commission basis or doctor or specialist visits require no interviews or background checks. This affects patient safety and the suitability of the healthcare professional is not confirmed. They are simply hired based on the urgent need for healthcare professionals all around.

Benefits of an Enterprise Hiring Solution

The proposed hiring system is a one stop integrated approach to getting the right persons for the right job and it is simple and automated partially to reduce travel and minimize costs.

Proposed solution

A new hiring system after all deliberations has been identified as follows consisting of an advertisement, selection, external online exams and training and final hiring with background checks and posting them to projects most of it conducted online with very fewer personal staff involvement.

How the proposed solution meets the requirement.

The proposed system has all the objectives required for hiring. The online application process will collect all the resumes and hiring managers will have access to the profiles to select candidates matching the projects the company has.

After they select the candidates, they can forward the shortlisted ones to the online exam agency to narrow down them to final selection and then hiring through personal video interviews online.

Selection of candidates

After receiving all the application forms either through print, advertisements or online, some will be shortlisted through a selection of the candidates within our internal HR department.

The most suitable candidates will be selected as applicable for the posts. A hiring agency having its own dedicated website will be involved in the interview process which will basically serve for giving online exams and identifying the right candidates out of the shortlisted profiles. (Dan Erling, 2010)

Training and online exam agency

An external training agency ABY will be involved in the interview process. This agency has its own dedicated online software system which has the necessary software allowing the candidates to give an exam online and selects the candidates automatically who pass the exam.

Some of the process is manual which includes an online video interview and post video interview selection of the final candidates and a training camp for the selected candidates.

The agencies selected have the necessary facilities for giving an online exam through internet anywhere in the world which eliminates the need to travel for giving exams.

Background check and screening

The background check requires the following information from the selected persons:

1. Completed I-9 form.

2. Copy of the Social Security Card.

3. Identity Photo ID a driving license, passport etc.

4. Signature on Offer of Letter.

5. A signed application form to be filled with all personal

details of employees and new employee/hire

information.

6. Welcome letter or appointment letter and joining letter on after the professional has joined work. This will be sent online through email after completion of all formalities.

CONCLUSION

The implementation part includes the narrowing down the selection of employees for our projects to the persons who have been selected in the final exams and submitting all the required documentation which comes in the implementation part.

Since the requirements are occasional and need based, these selected persons will for the final basis for recruitments as and when the needs arise provide, they fulfill all the conditions which essentially performance-based hiring. (Lou Adler, 2013)

There will be involvement of all the staff as mentioned in Stage 3 of the hiring process. The Company head may choose to get involved in the hiring process a need basis. He will be provided with information related to the hiring recommendation before making an offer to the selected persons. All applications are can be handled online if physical presence is not possible, to minimize communication and travel.

Chapter 12: Insurance and claims

ETHICS ALSO NEED TO be followed where the treatment is being carried out and not shown on paper as it happens in some cases. Professionals and patients have been found to take advantage of insurance by third party payers and faking and inflating costs to claims.

This issue needs to be addressed seriously and the healthcare professionals must work in the best interests of the patient, organization and third-party payers while evaluating such cases.

These practices have resulted in the redundancy if the mechanisms of accountability that were once appropriate to a health care system and for this reason the U.S. health system now considers the objectives of corporate management, shareholders, and the investment community through newer regulations.

Due to over inflated claims by hospitals, the insurance companies now do not cover the entire costs of treatments. Due to this the hospitals inflate the cost even further considering the reduction given by the insurance company. If the insurance company is paying only 70-80 percent the hospitals inflate costs to match the reduction.

Then in turn the insurance company increases the premiums on the policies resulting in more hardships to those having medical insurance.

For example, if the insurance premium was 50 dollars some years back, now patient pay 100 to 150 dollars for the same amount of coverage for treatment. Therefore, while insurance premium increases, so does the costs of treatment are artificially inflated as insurance companies instead of asking hospitals to reduce costs of treatments give only part claims.

The right process would have been to ask the hospital to charge a reasonable amount to the patient (the real customer in a Mediclaim is the insurance company). Had this been the case the cost of medical treatment would not increase year after year.

Patients need to insist for full coverage of medical costs and in many cases the medicines used are also over inflated. The unused medicines and bandages and other items are sent back to the medical stores which are often inhouse and excess medicines are recommended for purchase which are recycled back to the stores to be sold to another patients. This checking can only be done by the insurance companies and even for them it is not always

possible unless they have local representatives to check the claims properly.

This will help to avoid over inflated cost of treatment and only actual costs will be involved. This will act as a barrier for further increase in treatment costs which happen from time to time.

Chapter 13: Diagnostic testing

THE DISADVANTAGES OF diagnostic testing are the cost and treatments involved and the emotional setbacks if a certain disease is confirmed or positive making people feel guilty or unsafe.

We will study a few examples in this chapter to get an idea how diagnostic testing works and if it is beneficial or harmful and the risks involved.

Science is the study of how the universe works and humans have built scientific knowledge to develop technologies and make life easier and as technologies scientists are able to answer questions more than before.

Scientists have been able to understand the physics of visible light and its changes, when it passes through different mediums and used it to design microscopes.

Using microscopes, we were able to discover things which were not visible to the human eye. Biotechnology is important to the modern world to handle a growing population, poverty, fighting disease and protecting the environment.

Biotechnology is of two types, classical biotechnology and new biotechnology.

Classical biotechnology utilizes the natural chemical potential of cells or enzymes and has many industrial uses and in new biotechnology we produce genetically engineered cells. Both the terms come under the general term to describe the functioning of genetic engineering and related techniques. (US Congress, Office of Technology Assessment, 1984) .

Fermentation, brewing beer, baking of bread and breeding of animals existed even before cell phones came and did not require electricity or batteries, electric circuit boards, receivers, speakers, and satellites.

It has existed since prehistoric times and human beings realized that they could plant their own crops and breed animals, ferment juice into wince and convert milk into cheese or yogurt and ferment malt and hops which is in fact biotechnology.

The animal breeders mated appropriate pairs of animals and engaged in the manipulations of biotechnology. Biotechnology means different things to different people. For some it is developing new types of animals and for others, sources of human therapeutic drugs. Another possibility is growing nutritious and naturally pest-resistant plants. (Peters, 1993)

Biotechnology modifies cells of living organisms or their products to ferment alcoholic beverages, bacterial cells to make cheese and yogurts and make cows produce more milk for the same amount of feed. (Clark, Pazdernik, 2015)

The fermentation process allowed our ancestors to produce foods, by allowing live organisms to act on other ingredients and they found by manipulating the conditions of fermentation took place both quality and yield could be improved.

During fermentation microorganisms such as bacteria and yeast mix with ingredients that provide them food and they digest the food to produce carbon dioxide and alcohol.

Process of genetic testing

This includes testing genes in the laboratory which are the DNA instructions which we inherit from our parents. Genetic tests help to identify health problems and to select proper treatments or identify responses to treatments.

They also help to diagnose disease and to identify gene changes responsible for the disease and determine its severity. These results help doctors to decide the medicines required for the treatment and identify the genes that could pass on to children. New born babies can also be screened for genetic changes for certain treatments.

The gene changes are difficult to understand, and it gives information about your DNA, and may have implications for blood relatives. (Wolfe, 2015)

Types of genetic tests

Diagnostic testing: to identify the disease affecting the person.

Predictive and pre-symptomatic genetic tests: find gene changes that increase likelihood of a disease.

Carrier testing: for finding people who carry signs of genetic changes that may carry disease or an inherited disease belonging to certain groups that have a higher risk of inherited diseases.

Prenatal testing" is used during pregnancy.

Newborn screening: for new born babies.

Pharma-cogenetic testing: Identify how certain medicines affect people.

Research genetic testing: Research on links of genes to health and disease.

Advantage and disadvantages of genetic testing

Genetic testing eliminates the uncertainty regarding the health of a person and proves beneficial in the long-term giving more information on their health and it helps doctors select the treatments required. This can also help people decide about their future or their children's future by deciding to have babies or not. There are numerous benefits of early warning, dangers exist for persons undergoing the test and it may benefit others.

Counseling is needed and testing may be inappropriate for children and some other categories such as old aged people for whom knowing the information may be sensitive and hurtful.

All tests are not beneficial and for women who inherent mutations such as from BRAC1 and BRAC2, screening procedures, including self-examination, examination by a doctor, or a mammography, disease may still develop, and the outcome may not improve. For some tests are anxiety provoking and for some it is an essential requirement. (Smith, Quaid et al, 1998)

Angry, anxious or depressed and lead to discrimination in society. Genetic testing has limitations and cannot tell everything about inherent diseases. And a positive result does not necessarily mean a treatment can be done. The cost varies, anything between to a few hundred dollars to thousands depending on the diagnosis done.

Cloning

Genes are also cloned, and researchers use cloning to make identical copies. They insert genes from one organism a foreign DNA into a carrier such as bacteria, yeast or virus under laboratory conditions resulting in the multiplication of the genes.

Cloning humans and other animals much more difficult and cloning is expensive, and it will take years before we can have a high milk production and other benefits of cloning. Cloned animals face the difficulty of survival and liver, brain and heart. However, embryonic stem cells, have been used to generate almost all types of cells in an organism, to grow healthy tissues to replace injured tissues. (Brown, 2016)

Conclusion

Cloning affects our religious beliefs and society values and it conflicts with long standing issues as to who existed or will exist. If the human embryos used for testing are not destroyed, they may be used for wrongful purposes to collect embryonic stem cells. Therefore, I am totally opposed to cloning and stem cell research.

Other common issues affecting health care and the patients have been the high costs of health care and the payers, which may also be third party insurance companies are more than less willing to take on the burden of various procedures.

There is a scarcity of resource allocation decisions both by managers and physicians, and with limited financial, technical and knowledge resources, equitable and appropriate distribution has become necessary.

Mammogram and breast cancer testing

Breast cancer ranks next to lung cancer and there are more than a million breast cancer cases in women worldwide and causes large scale deaths USA, UK and Canada as well as other countries. The disease mostly occurs in women in the age group of 40 to 50 years and it is very important to detect it at an early stage.

Mammogram testing is required for females between the age of 40 and 50 and should ideally start at 40 years of ages. This diagnosis is used for testing for Cancer. X-rays are not safe mammogram also, due to the inherent risks associated with radiation.

But now we see doctors taking X-rays of young children, so it should be safe to take diagnosis with mammograms, and the benefits outweigh the risks. Identification of Cancer is important and the earlier we find out about it the treatments can start early and we can stay healthier.

Treatments for Cancer differ according to age groups, the earlier the treatment the less the medicines required. Accuracy of the testing is very important in testing with mammograms and all tests do not have 100 % accuracy. (Johnson, 2016)

Reynolds, 2016 notes that mammography introduced in the early 1970's, women face confusion for doing a mammogram, including health policy makers, and decisions regarding during mammography's initial launch made it all but inevitable that the test would be contentious.

The survival rates for breast cancer patients increase if the disease is detected at an early stage and assessment should include clinical, physical examination and an ultrasound. (Saunders, 2012)

A study of 179 samples at the Radiology Department Hospital, Sains University, Malaysia produced accuracy, sensitivity and specificity of 97%, 96% and 92% respectively for MAMMEX and it was 99%, 98% and 100% for SOUNDEX. The Receiver Operating Characteristics (ROC) curve analysis produced an Area Under the Curve (AUC) had values of 0.997 (±0.003) for MAMMEX and it was 0.996 (±0.004) for SOUNDEX. The Fuzzy-Count Image Processing (FCIP) and Automated Modified Seed-Based Region Growing (AMSBRG) techniques also facilitate the detection of micro calcifications.

Mammograms also give a false positive result and there are several opinions, making the women believe that mammograms are useful, but it is not so true. Death rates from breast cancer are the same even after a mammogram had been done, and mammograms are not as effective as it is believed. (Johnson, 2016).

The harmful effects of testing and tests and treatments that are performed after a false positive, are very dangerous and doctors cannot distinguish between dangerous and safe cancers. These tests are required and the probability that you have cancer is only 32%, and having tests exposes us to radiations.

The association of Body Mass Index (BMI) with Breast Cancer (BC) is important, but the exact effect of nonlinear dose-response for BMI and BC risk is not clear.

Obesity does contribute to increased BC risk in a nonlinear dose-response manner in post-menopausal women, and body weight control is crucial to reduce BC susceptibility. Some epidemiological studies suggest that obesity contribute to increased incidence of human cancer, including breast cancer (BC), and in view of this more attention should be paid to this obesity health problem, and newer approaches should be used to tackle the problems. (Xia, Chen, Li et. al., 2014)

Chapter 14: Child development observation and parental care

CHILDCARE SERVICES have become an important part of healthcare systems and starting from diagnosis of pregnancy and birth, lots of advancements have taken place in childcare development from infant to full growth.

Children need support either at the time of birth at the hospital or after discharge at the homes. Human babies are a dependent organism and depend on the parental care for growth in the first few years. They develop into full humans and further contribute to socioeconomic change and make significant progress in their domains as discussed in the Pals daycare video.

The Pals daycare video shows three infants in a caregiver site. These infants are given a wooden clothes pin and a plastic bottle, and the pin are to be placed inside the plastic bottle. While the first child drops the clothes pin on the floor and the other infants try to put the pin in the plastic bottle.

In this example the second child holds onto the pin and the third one tries to place the pin in the bottle. The third child has three wooden pins, so the caregiver takes away the other two and leaves the infant with one pin which it tries to place in the plastic bottle but fails.

This example shows that with the help of caregivers, children make inroads into self-development and social change and understand language as well as develop physical and motor development. The basic needs of the infant are attended to through proper care and attention. The infants in the Pals daycare video are learning to hold the pins in their hands and place them inside the plastic bottle.

The cognitive development takes place when the first infant uses his hands, mouth and touch sensation to feel the wooden pins and the second infant manages to hold the pin in his hand which is the second stage of development. The third stage of development is exemplified by the third infant who tries to place the wooden pin inside of the plastic bottle.

The first infant is also watching the activities of the other two infants as they try to place their wooden pins inside the plastic bottles individually which shows the development of observation.

Cognitive development depends on the five senses of smell, touch, vision, taste and hearing and the infants tried to use these five senses to experiment with placing the wooden pin inside of the plastic bottle. (Bigner, 2009).

Language and communication are used through being expressive or through gestures and the infant use sound to communicate with each other as well as with the parental caregiver. Here in the video the infants babble some words to the caregiver and make expressions.

Using reflexes, the physical and motor development takes place. The handling and placing of the wooden pin are an example of the physical and motor development during the infant stage of development using their hands and arms.

The social and emotional development takes place through laughing and smiling and feeling happy. Some are alert while others are silent and watching and paying attention to the environment around them. (Santrock, 2009). There is trust in the caregiver and the infant even smiles in front of the camera.

In the observation first the infant tried to hold on to the wooden pin and he dropped the pin even after the caregiver tried to help him.

The first infant the watched the other infants who were more successful in holding on to the pin to learn from them. This type of child development is encouraged, and the use of toys is very much like this idea which helps the child develop socially as well as emotionally.

Toys and games help in motor and physical development. Nursery rhymes and songs are another medium which help in using sound in child development.

With more and more focus of people on work and earning money the time needed to spend on a child has become limited and many parents rely on caregivers to take care of their children. The children become more attached to the caregivers rather than the parents and this is an important challenge for future parents.

Also, now children must rely more on television and toys and other learning techniques which were earlier taught by parents. But since parents are busy in work and the focus on both husband and wife working, the attention on children is limited.

Children suffer illnesses without the knowledge of the parents who are too busy in work or socializing and are not admitted into hospitals until something seriously happens. The days when children were sent for a regular checkup at hospitals have become limited due to more importance on treating adult patients.

Children are expected more to self-recover and take-home based medicines or over the counter products. They are not even attended by nurses seriously as patients even when admitted in hospitals and when they complain of an illness, it is taken as an excuse for skipping school or colleges.

These smaller illnesses then grow into big ones and then require major treatments. Schools and colleges have access to doctors, but the illness is often hidden as disclosing would mean the child being dismissed from school or loss in studies.

Other problems would include other children avoiding a child diagnosed with a disease with the excuse that they would also contract the same.

The healthcare system should convince other children that when doctors and other staff do not contract diseases of the patients it is not possible for once child to get diseased from another for most of the diseases except those spread through in some cases.

Awareness must be created in the school and college levels which will lower the burden at the time of adulthood. In some cases, the parents are sick, and the children are too young to look after them and these are also some of the challenges faced in healthcare.

In underdeveloped countries there are many NGOs working for providing treatment to children and elderly patients. But even after so much resource allocation, there is a problem in getting funds for treatment. While patients get admitted in hospitals, they have no money to pay bills.

The healthcare industry earns a lot of money through treatment, diagnostic testing as visits by doctors and specialists, but it has never contributed in return to provide a percentage of their earnings to treat the needy and the poor and children admitted in hospitals except for a very few rare cases.

Those few who help are shown in newspapers and magazines in headlines and get immense popularity for helping some needy patient which shows how few people are present in the industry to offer help to some of the patients who have no finance source to pay for treatments.

While it is not always possible to help who all are in need, there can be alternatives like reducing costs of treatment, finding government support etc. While NGOs are ready to help but they lack funds and the funds they collect always seem to be insufficient as they target funds from the lower- and middle-class people.

The major reason is that the rich and affluent feel that they have ample resources for their own treatments and will not require an NGO help plus they also have Mediclaim as a backup. Therefore, the premium and rich class do not contribute significantly to the NGOs as they feel it is not necessary to support them as they may or may not require help of an NGO in future.

This mindset needs to be changed so more funds can come from an affluent class of people which can pay and claim tax benefits offered by contributing for such causes.

Notes

TECHBAGG@OUTLOOK.COM

Don't miss out!

Click the button below and you can sign up to receive emails whenever Jagdish Krishanlal Arora publishes a new book. There's no charge and no obligation.

Sign Me Up!

https://books2read.com/r/B-A-XQZZ-MTCVC

BOOKS 2 READ

Connecting independent readers to independent writers.

Did you love *Productive Healthcare Management*? Then you should read *How to Lose Weight Quickly* by Jagdish Krishanlal Arora!

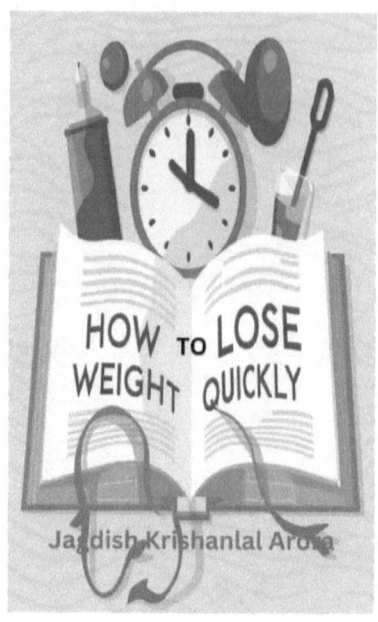

Losing weight is often not recommended for sustained and healthy weight management. However, adopting a combination of strategies such as following a balanced and reduced-calorie diet, increasing physical activity levels, staying adequately hydrated, managing stress, ensuring sufficient sleep, and avoiding processed foods and sugary beverages can support initial weight loss. It's important to prioritize gradual and sustainable changes to foster long-term success, rather than opting for rapid weight loss methods that may compromise overall health and result in regaining weight in the long run.

Also by Jagdish Krishanlal Arora

Basic Inorganic and Organic Chemistry
Book of Jokes
Car Insurance and Claims
Digital Electronics, Computer Architecture and Microprocessor Design Principles
Guided Meditation and Yoga
The Bible and Jesus Christ
Unity Quest
From Oasis to Global Stage: The Evolution of Arab Civilization
Secrets of Mount Kailash, Bermuda Triangle and the Lost City of Atlantis
Visitors from Outer Space
Motivation
The Aliens and God Theory
The Lunar Voyager
Queen Elizabeth II and the British Monarchy
The Kremlin Conspiracy
Vegetable Gardening, Salads and Recipes
How to End The War in Ukraine
The Old and New World Order
Stellaris
Travelling to Mars in the Cosmic Odyssey 2050
Romance Pays Off
How the Universe Works
Mental Health and Well Being
Ancient History of Mars
The Nexus
Basic and Advanced Physics
Administrative Law
Calculus
The Ramayana
A Watery Mystery

Romantic Conflicts
Thieves of Palestine
Love in Chicago
WordPress Design and Development
Travellers Guide to Mount Kailash
Become a Better Writer With Creative Writing
Emerging Trends in Carbon Emission Reduction
India Independence Through Non Violence
Copyright, Patents, Trademarks and Trade Secret Laws
Decoding CHATGPT and Artificial Intelligence
The Untold Story of Diana and Prince Charles
Time Travel
How to Lose Weight Quickly
Subconcious Programming
Productive Healthcare Management

www.ingramcontent.com/pod-product-compliance
Lightning Source LLC
Chambersburg PA
CBHW021509210526
45463CB00002B/960